THE PREHISTORIC DIET

(For the Modern Man and Woman)

20 MILLION YEARS IN THE MAKING

J. ALEXANDER

Order this book online at www.trafford.com
or email orders@trafford.com

Most Trafford titles are also available at major online book retailers.

Printed in Victoria, BC, Canada.

ISBN: 978-1-4269-1931-2

Trafford rev. 11/23/2009

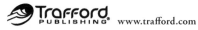 www.trafford.com

North America & international
toll-free: 1 888 232 4444 (USA & Canada)
phone: 250 383 6864 ♦ fax: 812 355 4082

ACKNOWLEDGEMENTS

I want to thank my wonderful children, Daniel, Brooke and Benjamin for supporting my endeavor.

To my Mom Ethel, thank you for initially instilling within me the need to "think outside of the box" when it comes to the Natural ways of healing vs. needelsss medications.

My great appreciation to my front book designer Lauren A. Linden for her input and dedication.

The interpretation of her front cover art being "Who we were and who we can be."

Many thanks to Benjamin Linden, my chief editor for his terrific and devoted work.

Contents

1

Why I Wrote This Book

"If I am not for myself, who will be for me? And if I am only for myself, what am I? And if not now, when?"

-Rabbi Hillel

Look over your shoulder; your childhood is following you. Our parents were wonderful, hardworking, loving— and clueless about nutrition.

In the days of *Lassie*, *Mouseketeers*, and *Happy Days* our diets were composed primarily of heavy meats, starches such as mashed white potatoes, pastas (many from a can), Chinese food (also from a can), white bread (nice and smooth) and mixed powdered sweet drinks. Cooked vegetables were cooked…and cooked…and cooked to a nice mushy consistency while the so-called salad consisted of overripe tomatoes, lettuce (which, it was made sure, was not so crisp as to take on the same consistency as the tomatoes), maybe a radish (which was purely for color

1

since no one ate it) and—thank goodness—a heavy salad dressing to manage an attempt at a salad. We had fish on the "off day" almost as a punishment, but things got better once battered fish sticks were invented.

Of course, for breakfast we had our multicolored and heavenly and heavily sweetened cereals or French toast, which had to be made with smooth white bread with no holes, and with lots of fake maple syrup and butter. Mom had a deep freezer so we could help ourselves to desserts a plenty—pies, ice cream, popsicles, and fudgesicals.

Fruit? Oh, we had our orange concentrate and a couple of apples that no one dared to approach because of their sad expressions. And when it came to sodas we had them with nice pure sugars and syrups since diet soda wasn't really an option then.

My childhood eating habits were really not that much different than those of millions of American households today, except that I did not have the thousands of fast food options that we have today, and the foods we ate then did not have the numerous "new and improved" additives that foods have today, many of which most of us don't have a clue how to say, much less define. Take the following additives I found on a box of cereal: polydextrose, coconut and palm kernel oils, cocoa processed with alkali, and BHA (butylated hydroxyanisole), plus artificial flavors (why do we even need them?). And why in another cereal do we need modified cornstarch, trisodium phosphate, and calcium carbonate?

As a child I became heavy or chubby, but not obese. My parents and siblings somehow stayed slim. Socially I felt unpopular; I was certainly not the athletic type and certainly not happy. Again, I was not obese but certainly stood out as the object of ridicule, as did maybe two or three percent of my classmates who were also heavy— we were the "heavy clique". In addition, I had terrible allergies to almost everything so I was put on years of allergy injections and antihistamines, which made me groggy and slowed down my metabolism. These injections would often cause my arm to swell up and would always carry the possibility of causing me to go into shock. So the die was cast early on—I would always battle against extra weight and allergies.

At the age of 13, with a more expanded waist, Mom bought special "Curb Your Appetite" diet drinks, which I brought to the school lunchrooms to go along with saltine crackers, a hardboiled egg, and one of those very sad-looking apples. To this day I get a nauseous feeling thinking about this lunchtime cuisine. Meanwhile my classmates would sit down to their lunches of baloney-on-white-bread sandwiches with bags of potato chips and chocolate cupcakes and cola drinks. Well, at least my diet was a start, and I did take off some weight for a while until I went off that diet drink.

The battle continued and in my twenties I became convinced that natural foods were the answer. It was at this point that I opened one of the first that I opened "Food for Thought" one of the first health food stores in Boston Massachusetts. Working at the store was a wonderful learning experience since I observed so many of our customers being able to relieve themselves of so many ailments by educating themselves about the miracles of good, natural, unadulterated food. I myself was able to finally cease my weekly allergy injections, which, in reality, never seemed to help anyway. What did help was my understanding of which foods and environmental circumstances would trigger my allergies, hay fever and severe laryngitis and which foods and vitamins were beneficial.

Nevertheless, weight was always an issue for me. I did not try diet pills or expensive food programs since I knew of many people who tried and failed with these programs and who almost always put the weight back on—and sometimes ended up even heavier than before. Thanks to the PREHISTORIC DIET, extra weight and allergies are no longer issues for me. My life has changed for the better; I am now the person I was meant to be.

I wish I could say the same for the rest of the country. In today's America, the obesity statistics are staggering. We no longer see a slightly overweight person here and there. Instead, we are faced with an obesity rate of almost one in three. The Centers for Disease Control and Prevention found that the most Obese state is Mississippi with almost 33 percent obesity, while the least obese state is Colorado at just under 20 percent.[1] So congratulations to the great state of Colorado: only one in 5 is obese. Even though when I was in school it was no more than 3 out of 100 that was just heavy...

In reality, this is very bad news, and it greatly increases the crucial need to work out our country's obesity situation. A new study shows that some overweight teenagers have too much body fat, which results in severe liver damage. The study notes that "a handful has needed liver transplants. Many more may need a new liver by the time they reach their 30's and 40's," and "by 2020 experts predict fatty liver disease will become the number one cause of liver transplants." This disease is called "nonalcoholic fatty liver disease."[2]

According to The Centers For Disease Control, 72 million Americans are obese in a finding from 2005-2006.[3] My guess is that as of 2009 it must be even higher. Jack Rosemarin M.D., F.A.C.G., notes that 300,000 Americans die each year due to complications of obesity-related diseases such as colon cancer, heart disease, arthritis, type-two diabetes, high blood pressure, liver disease and pre-cancerous polyps. In addition, other ailments related to obesity include gall bladder disease, sleep apnea, respiratory problems, infertility, depression, back problems, stroke, varicose veins, fatigue and more.

As I mentioned, your childhood follows you, and my empathy for our obese children is very passionate. At the rate America's eating habits are going, our children are condemned to lives of misery, hardship and disease.

Our politicians and leaders talk about the high cost of health care in front of audiences that are at least a third obese, with canes to assist their heavy bodies to walk, and who can hardly get off the chair to applaud when the speaker is done. The politician will never mention to them (because it is not politically correct) that one of the main reasons—if not *the* main reason—for the high health care costs is that many of their constituents are just too darn fat.

Yes, many European countries as well as Japan and many other countries in the developed world have wonderful universal healthcare coverage, but please note that the populations of these counties are for the most part trim and fit, and therefore don't have to deal with the huge list of obesity-related ailments. They are thus spared from the huge expenses associated with massive obesity.

Recently I had a disturbing observation when I visited in the hospital a patient with a heart condition.

Well over 75% of the patients I noticed throughout the hospital and the hospital staff were either very overweight or obese.

A nurse who was advising a patient on Diet was herself quite overweight.

The hospital cafeteria was loaded with greasy foods, pasteries, sodas, and very few fruits and vegetables.

I noticed hospital staff (Obese) devouring greasy cheeseburgers, bags of potato chips, giant sodas and deserts.

If this is the general situation in our "Hospitals" what could be more indicative of the Diet/Obesity problem we have in our nation.

How can the Obese advise those with heart disease and other Obesity/bad food related ailments.

No wonder our health costs are so high.

I felt like I was in Alice in Wonderland..all rationale being upside down..

I am quite certain if I were observing hospitals in parts of Europe and Japan the hospital staff would be trim, healthier and highly credible.

According to a report by the Office of the U.S. Surgeon General, in the year 2000, the direct and indirect health care costs of obesity to the United States were $117 billion. Now in 2009 the costs are bound to be much higher.

And so for our children (and the rest of us) I wrote this book.

2

No, I Will Not Put *That* Stuff into *My Body*

The damage that fast foods do to our bodies has been thoroughly documented, so it's a given that if you wish to lose weight and live a healthier lifestyle, fast foods are a BIG FAT NO. Many people desperately hope the modern marketed "diet food plans" will do it, but the fact is that they usually don't. One may spend a lot of time and money on these plans. It's well documented that while you may initially lose some weight, the weight eventually comes back after you finish the plan (which is marketed to be only a temporary plan), often worse than before.

Many users are also unaware of the ingredients used in these "Diet Food Plans", many of which are highly suspect. First, let's take a look at those diet drinks and the energy drinks that are sold primarily in cans and plastic bottles:

The Cans and Bottles Themselves:

"The U.S. Centers for Disease Control and Prevention have documented widespread exposure to a variety of chemicals, including bisphenol-A, found in hard plastics and the lining of cans."[1]

"Bisphenal-A is a hormone disrupter that is also used in dental sealants and in the resins that line cans."[2]

"Studies with rodents have shown that exposure to high doses of bisphenol-A during pregnancy and/or lactation can reduce survival birthrate and growth of off-spring early in life and delay the onset of puberty in males and females"[3]

The National Toxicology Program and an expert panel has noted "some concern that the exposure to bisphenol-A in utero causes neural and behavioral effects," "minimal concern that exposure to bisphenol A in utero causes effects on the prostate," "minimal concern that exposure to Bisphenol A in utero potentially causes accelerations in puberty," and "negligible concern that exposure to Bisphenal-A in utero produces birth defects and malformations."[4] Why should we accept even minimal or negligible risks to our health when it comes to what we drink? We should be able to drink what we want to without *any* fear of poisoning.

Energy Drinks

For those seeking weight loss, some feel that with an energy drink they will be able to pursue more exercise. Indeed, the market for these drinks has grown at a rapid pace. These drinks are advertised as being nutritious and some do contain vitamins and herbal extracts. The main ingredients, however, are LOTS of sugar and caffeine.

Nutritionist Dee Rollins with Baylor University says that she is aware of over 200 energy drinks on the market and notes that "some of these energy drinks contain a couple of hundred milligrams of caffeine per one drink." Many drink manufacturers don't advertise the amount of caffeine in their drinks and Rollins warns about taking too much of this powerful central-nervous system stimulant. She explains that 250 milligrams a day is what is considered safe in the United States while a level of 300 milligrams is often considered excessive. Some of these energy drinks contain over 200 milligrams of caffeine in one bottle, meaning that drinkers are nearly exceeding their safe daily limit in one can or bottle of energy drink. A single cup of coffee, by contrast, contains between 80-120 milligrams of caffeine. Rollins says that the symptoms of too much caffeine in a day can lead to nervousness, headaches, increased heart rate and higher blood pressure, depression, poor concentration and insomnia.[5]

Some of these drinks contain a substance called D-ribose which is "a five-compound sugar...and there is no credible evidence that it is an effective energizer." This substance, when consumed in excess, can lead to weight gain. In addition, there are about two teaspoons of sugar per eight-ounce can in many of these energy drinks.[6]

Diet sodas

It seems to me that when observing who is drinking diet soft drinks, a great number are obese. Months after observing the same people, they are still obese. These are diet sodas that are marketed as an aid in weight loss, but I have not heard of anyone who has lost weight by drinking diet soda. Have you?

While I am certainly NOT a proponent of *any* sodas, I do feel that non-diet sodas are a bit preferable to the diet ones. My personal feeling is that the body is not able to cope with all the additives in the diet drinks, and that these additives retard the body's ability to eliminate fat.

According to studies by Dr. Vasan Ramachandran of the Boston University School of Medicine, "diet sodas are linked to heart disease risks more so than those that drink regular sugared sodas." Diet drinks may also increase the craving for more sweets. One or more diet or regular soda per day has been shown to increase the risk of metabolic syndrome—a cluster of symptoms that increase the risk of heart attack and often lead to larger waistlines as well as higher levels of blood pressure, blood sugar, cholesterol, and blood fats called triglycerides. One or more drinks a day amount to a 44% higher chance of metabolic syndrome.

People who drink large amounts of sweetened drinks are prone to developing a taste for sweetened foods since the substance that gives soda its caramel color promotes resistance to insulin, which is needed to process calories."[7]

Additives

I will now review a listing of some of the additives found in most diet drinks. After reading about the possible negative side effects of these additives, I believe that you too will agree that they should be avoided.

Aspartame:

At the World Environmental Conference, it was suggested that aspartame has devastating effects on the body. Marketed as *NutraSweet, Equal,* and *Spoonful,* aspartame is found in most if not all diet sodas (and is also used in over 6,000 diet products). Symptoms such as fibromyalgia, spasms, shooting pains, numbness of the legs, cramps, vertigo, seizures, dizziness, headaches, tinnitus (ringing in the ears), joint pain, depression, anxiety attacks, slurred speech, blurred vision, and memory loss were noted with aspartame consumption.

Some doctors believe that poisoning from aspartame mimics multiple sclerosis, sometimes leading to misdiagnosis. Systemic lupus is believed to be another misdiagnosis from this aspartame poisoning. Doctors are finding relief of symptoms when patents are removed from aspartame, yet it is still on the market.

Birth defects such as mental retardation have also been linked to aspartame poisoning and lab tests using aspartame have resulted in brain tumors in animals.[8]

At the Cancer Research Center in Bologna Italy, aspartame was fed to rats with the "results showing that aspartame in our experimental conditions cause a statistically significant related increase in lymphomas and leukemias in females."[9] There has also been research done linking aspartame to brain tumors.[10] Amazingly, the Food and Drug Administration has acknowledged 92 symptoms of aspartame poisoning.[11] Why, then, is it still on the market?

Some diet drinks contain Phenylalanine, which is fifty percent aspartame. Janet Starr Hull, creator of the Aspartame Detox Program, notes that "too much phenylalanine is a neurotoxin and excites the neutrons on the brain to the point of cellular death. ADD/ADHD, emotional and behavioral disorders can all be triggered by too much Phenylalanine in the daily diet".[12]

Additionally, aspartame "could cause aspartame disease... [which] consists of cramps, vertigo, headaches, depression, [and] memory loss, among other ailments. Byproducts of aspartame are methanol formaldehyde and are also found in fruit juices," (not the natural fruit juices but those that are processed). It has been noted that "aspartame can be related to depression and bipolar disorders".[13]

During 2001, "Senator Howard Metzenbaum wrote a bill that would have instituted independent studies (on aspartame), but it was squelched by the powerful food, drug, and chemical companies."

Please note the following warning from the Consumer Science Protection Institute (CSPI), dated June 25 2007: "As a result of a new study the Ramazzini Foundation/ CSPI is warning consumers 'Everyone should avoid aspartame.'" In a new study published in the Journal *Environmental Health Perspectives*, The Ramazzini Foundation found that aspartame significantly increases lymphomas and leukemia in rats, while another study published in January 2007 shows that it also alters the genes in animals. The report from the CSPI also states that in a study at the Institute of Public Health at the University of Pecs, Hungary, aspartame caused lymphomas, brain tumors and transitional cell tumors.

On April 17, 2007, "*Sainsbury,* Britain's third-largest supermarket, announced they will be removing aspartame sweetener from its private-label soft drinks." Meanwhile, on April 23, 2007, Dr. Morando Soffrith of the European Ramazzini Foundation presented results of a new study confirming the carcinogenicity of aspartame at Mt. Sinai Medical School of New York.[14]

Citric Acid:

It has been reported that ingestion of large amounts of citric acid may cause vomiting and diarrhea and other gastrointestinal disturbances. It may also contribute to calcium deficiencies.[15]

High Fructose Corn Syrup:

This is a sweetener that over a period of time will damage your pancreas.

Phosphoric Acid:

Over a period of time erodes the enamel on your teeth.[16]

Phosphates:

A study in South Korea found that when added to foods, organic phosphates strongly assisted the development of lung cancer in mice. Myung-Haing Cho of the Seoul National University, who led the study, noted that a diet high in phosphates "significantly increased the lung surface tumor lesions as well as the size."[17] Phosphates are also found in processed meats, cheeses, and baked goods.

Caramel Color:

This food coloring is made by heating food-grade carbohydrates, and is generally "a high dextrose containing starch hydrolyzed or corn syrup acids such as acetic acid, lactic acid, or phosphoric acid which may be used to break the bonds between sugars before the sugars are raised to a higher temperature for carmelization."[18] In other words, more acids and sugars.

Diet Foods/Diet Food Systems

Now let's take a look at the diet foods and diet food systems that we constantly hear so much about on television commercials and in all other forms of media. When it comes to these foods, here are the facts:

1. They usually don't taste all that good.

2. They are expensive.

3. While you may lose weight at first, statistics show that most users put back on the weight and often add more, leading many to just give up.

4. Many of the ingredients are highly suspect when it comes to health benefits and nutritional value.

Here are just a few of the ingredients that I find worrisome (to say the least):

Methyl Cellulose:

Manufactured in China, a powdery substance prepared synthetically by methylation of natural cellulose and used as a food additive, a bulk-forming laxative, an emulsifier and thickener, that swells in water to form a gel.[19]

Hydrogenated Corn Oil:

Hydrogenated oils are fats that have the same capacity to do harm as saturated fats. They also pose another health hazard: trans fatty acids. The trans fats significantly raise the bad cholesterol levels while lowering the good cholesterol levels, which is the cause of coronary heart disease.

Hydrogenation extends the supermarket shelf life[20] (but certainly does not extend our lives). Hydrogenated oils are proven to be a cause of type-two diabetes, cancer, autism, food allergies, and autoimmune diseases. Some studies show that there is a 40 percent increase in Breast Cancer in women who eat hydrogenated oils.[21]

Sodium Aluminum Phosphate:

In a study, men were fed biscuits containing aluminum phosphate in addition to normal dietary items. Blood and urine samples were taken two, four, six, and eight hours after the meal. Aluminum was frequently found in their blood. The results of the Aluminum rich diet caused occasional slight increase of aluminum in the blood and also in the urine.[22] Aluminum antacids may cause inhibition of the intestinal absorption of phosphorus and then cause calcium loss.[23]

Fructose Corn Syrup:

"Unused amounts are stored as fat cells. Instead of burning this energy, sedentary kids store more and more of it and because of this they are getting fatter." Meira Fields, a research chemist at USDA in Beltsville Maryland, notes that "rats usually live a good 2 years. Rats fed high fructose, low copper diets are dying after 5 weeks." Fields continues, "high fructose diets have also been implicated in the development of adult onset diabetes. Meanwhile, Richard Anderson, a leading scientist at the Human Nutrition Research Center in Beltsville Maryland, notes that "Fructose, especially when combined with other sugars, reduces stores of chromium, a mineral essential for maintaining balanced insulin levels."[24]

Sodium Phosphate:

Usually used as a drug and "should not be used if you have kidney disease, congestive heart failure, electrolyte imbalance and in sodium restricted diets. Toxicity may occur and could cause swelling in the face, lips, tongue or throat, and can cause stomach pain and nausea.[25]

Caramel Color:

Also a sugary substance (see section on diet sodas).

Potassium Chloride:

Potassium Chloride is used primarily in the production of fertilizer.[26] It should also be noted that "as a medication, you should not use potassium chloride if you have kidney failure, Addison disease, or if you are dehydrated.[27]

Dextrose:

A type of sugar.[28] Isn't it illogical for diet foods to have sugar added?

Vitamin A Palmitate:

A Synthetically produced chemical.[29]

Xanthan Gum:

Xanthan gum "derives it's name from the strain of bacteria used during fermentation process," and is derived from *xanthomonas campertris*, "the same bacteria responsible for causing black rot to form on broccoli and cauliflower. The bacteria form a slimy substance that puts a natural stabilizer or thickness on the *xanthomnas compestris* and is combined with corn sugar, resulting in xanthan gum. Some have complained of abdominal cramps and diarrhea. Some get hives and there have been reports of anaphyscitic shock.[30]

Guar Gum:

"In the late 1980's it was used and heavily promoted in several weight loss products. The USFDA eventually recalled these due to reports of esophageal blockage from insufficient fluid intake after one brand also caused ten hospitalizations and one death."[31]

Ferrous Sulfate:

It has been found to have "low toxicity in small quantities..." and can cause "aggravation of those with pre-existing condition of skin disorder, eye problems, kidney or respiratory functions"[32]

Cargeenan:

It has no nutrition value. Experiments with rats have show possible linkages to colon cancer.[33]

Malto Dextrin:

A carbohydrate made from natural cornstarch, which is well known to cause weight gain. Huh!! What is the rationale here?

Yeast Extract:

Dr. Russell Blaylock, author of *Excitotoxins*, notes that "for many people [yeast extract] has the same effect as MSG: migraine headaches, chemical taste enhancement and harm to the nervous system."[34]

Modified Corn Starch:

Starch is well known to cause weight gain and what is the rationale here?

Ferric Phosphate:

Used in fertilizer, medicines, and pesticides, it includes an active ingredient used to control snails and slugs.

There are other foreign elements used in these "Diet Foods" but I assume that by now you've come to ask yourself the same question I have: Why would anyone want these things in their body?

Nano-Foods

This is a new genetically engineered food that some consumers are fearful of. The process of producing nano-foods is used as a flavor enhancer that involves the design and manipulation of materials on molecular scales. Nano products are coming on the market at a rate of 4 per week. According to an advocacy group called *The Project on Emergency Nanotechnologies*, there are now over 600 nano-products.

Dr. Michael Hansen, a senior scientist with the Consumers Union notes that "recent studies have shown that nano-size particles in some cases can invade cells and breach the blood-brain barrier, and that some forms of nano-size carbon could be as harmful as asbestos if inhaled in [high quantities]." He continues, "these technologies raise basic scientific issues."[35]

Soy Products

We have been led to believe that soy products are nutritious, one of the most perfect forms of protein, a great replacement for dairy products, and a wonderful alternative for meat products. Basically, we have been led to believe that they are perfect for any diet. Unfortunately, I don't believe this to be true.

Many soy products are produced in factories, which in itself should make us suspicious of this supposedly natural food. In ancient Asia, soybean plantings were utilized as an agricultural soil product for crop rotation in order to put Nitrogen-13 back into the soil. For any benefits at all, soybean food products must be fermented. Tempe, miso, and soy sauce are examples of food products that are made out of fermented soy.

Unfermented soybeans contain large amounts of natural toxins such as potent enzyme inhibitors that block the action of trypsin and other enzymes needed for protein digestion. Diets that are high in trypsin inhibitors cause enlargement and pathological conditions of the pancreas, including cancer.[36] Soybeans also contain hemoglutinin, which is a clot-promoting substance that causes red blood cells to clump together. Trypsin inhibitors and hemoglutinin are also growth inhibitors. Soy also contains goitrogen, a substance that depress thyroid function.

99 percent of soybean products are genetically modified and have one of the highest percentages of

contamination by pesticides of any foods. Soybeans are high in phatic acid, which can block the uptake of essential minerals such as calcium, magnesium, copper, iron and zinc.

Scientists generally agree that grain and legume-based diets are high in "phytates" which contribute to widespread mineral deficiencies in third world countries.[37] In 1991, researches in Japan revealed that consumption of as little as 30 grams (2 teaspoons) of soybeans per day for only one month resulted in a significant increase in thyroid-stimulating hormones and diffuse goiter.[38]

It's our body. We must be our own advocate and the advocate of our love ones. We must be on guard as to what we admit into the sanctity of our bodies.

3

THE PREHISTORIC DIET
(Hello Adam, Hello Eve)

I have always had this GUT (no pun intended) feeling that if we ate as our prehistoric ancestors did then we would be much healthier. They certainly had to be a lot stronger since the sedentary life really wasn't much of an option. They therefore needed to obtain the optimum nutrition in order to survive. My rationale is that it took nature 20 million years of evolution in order to perfect our systems. Who are we to mess with nature's work?

For many thousands of years, early man had within his environment all the nutrients that nature took millions of years to create for him. All of these nutrients were, of course, unprocessed and were not cultivated since the Agricultural Revolution came only recently in man's history. So before Agriculture picture this:

"Gee Mom, I'm hungry!"

"Well dear, get out of the cave find yourself a treat and also be sure to pick up some groceries and bring them back for the family."

What "treats and groceries" were found? Our ancestors were hunter-gatherers so they went back home with raw nuts, beautiful fruits, mushrooms, and wild greens. If they had access to the ocean they would bring home seaweed, fish, and shellfish. There was wild poultry, eggs, mammoth to be hunted (burgers anyone?), along with bison (more burgers), deer and other game. There were lots of berries, wild herbs and many root vegetables, insects and other small creatures of the day.

Their drinking water was fresh. They did not nourish themselves with dairy products other than mother's milk, which provided them with nutrients that would last them a lifetime. When one ingests the milk of an animal is one also ingesting the toxins of the animal? Millions of people throughout the world today are lactose intolerant, which means the others can *tolerate* it. To *tolerate*, of course, does not mean to *need* it.

So, in a sense, the nutrition situation was perfect back then. Maybe, as the Bible tells us, man really was in the Garden of Eden. We've all seen those renditions of Adam and Eve: They looked marvelous. They were not obese, no huge buttocks or bellies, no canes or walkers or motorized chairs to assist walking or one's transport because of obesity. They were trim and beautiful. In sum, prehistoric man ate to live; he didn't live to eat.

Then one day, many of thousands of years ago, Adam and Eve picked that darn apple. Could that moment have been a metaphor for the beginning of the Agricultural Revolution? The bible mentions that they were banned from the Garden of Eden and from then on had to fend for themselves. In other words they had to work the land and cultivate and process new foods. The new foods were grains and dairy products.

Many Anthropologists agree through their research that with this Agricultural Revolution, man's nutrition started to decline. Bones and teeth were not as strong. In a sense, many of the food became "processed". Grains were cultivated and highly processed into breads and cakes. Dairy was consumed— more often from the beast than from the mother.

Then, around 1900 AD, man began embellishing on his use of dairy, grains and sugars by processing and refining them further, removing many of the nutrients (i.e. refined and bleached flour, rice and sugars). By the 1950's preservatives and additives used for various reasons were added to the foods and have been added continuously since. The result has been that nutrition from these so-called "foods" today is an absolute mess, resulting in the present obesity situation and all the complications that come with it.

According to Dr. S. Boyd Eaton, millions of years of evolution have shaped our needs for specific nutrients. "Modern diets are out of sync with our genetic requirements and the less we eat as our ancestors, the more susceptible you'll be to coronary disease, cancer, diabetes, and other modern diseases." He goes on, "ninety-nine percent of our genetic heritage dates from before our biological ancestors evolved into homosapiens around 40,000 years ago and 99.9 % of our genes were formed before the development of agriculture around 10,000 years ago."[1] Now, we no longer leave the cave for berries, nuts, etc., but instead go to our local "Junk Food" establishments for take out. Or maybe just have this "Stuff" delivered because we are to lazy or heavy to walk there.

Recently there was a study on those 20-40 years old. They were fed only fresh fruits, berries, vegetables (not legumes), fish and seafood (unsalted), lean meats, raw nuts (not peanuts, which are legumes), flaxseed or grape seed oil and lemon and lime juice as a salad dressing, coffee and tea (without sugar or dairy), and water. They were fed these foods for a 3-week period. After the three-week period here were some of the results:

- An average weight loss of 5 lbs.

- An average reduction of the waistline of ½".

- An average reduction of high blood pressure.

- A 72 percent reduction in the levels of a substance known as plasminogen activator inhibitor-1. This would be expected to reduce the clotting tendency of the blood, which might translate into a reduced risk of heart attack and stroke.

Regarding weight loss, Dr. John Briffa, London-based states, "when individuals move their diet in a primal direction, they very often end up eating less quite naturally and tend to shed weight with relative ease."[2]

I decided to get in touch with our Prehistoric Ancestral roots, and to eat as they did. I wanted to loose weight and to acquire any other additional benefits. In the next chapter we will discuss the numerous great foods we can take advantage of and their nutrient qualities. I'll go over my basic food intake, which is the basis of THE PREHISTORIC DIET. I'll also briefly discuss what foods to stay away from. In a subsequent chapter I will share with you some ideas for recipes. I assure you that once you get the hang of this miraculous diet, you too will be making up your own recipes.

Right now, however, I want to share with you some of the exciting results that I began to notice within 3 weeks of starting our ancestral diet. Here are *some* of those exciting results:

- I lost 13 pounds.

- I went from a 36-inch waist to a 32-inch waist.

- I am never hungry since I can eat as much as I want (from the Prehistoric Diet), whenever I want.

- I have much more energy, allowing me to spend some time doing basic exercises like push-ups, light weights, sit-ups and power walking.

- I have all around better body tone

- Sex is better than ever. Having more energy and more self esteem from the weight loss is very beneficial in this area.

Here are some additional observations on how an the Prehistoric Diet can improve one's sex life:

- "Chili Peppers and Ginger are believed to improve circulation and stimulate nerve endings, which in turn improve sexual pleasure."[3]

- "There has been solid research showing that obesity is a risk factor for erectile dysfunction and low testosterone," says Dr. Ridwan Shabsigh, director of the New York Center for Human Sexuality and associate Professor of Urology at Columbia University Medical School. "Reducing weight," he says, "results in an increase of the testosterone and thus an increase in sexual function."

- "You need fat to produce your hormones" says Beverly Whipple, Professor Emeritus at Rutgers University and President of the World Association of Sexology. "Cholesterol is metabolized in the liver, and you get your testosterone and estrogen which you need for your sex drive." Whipple goes on to say that olive oil, salmon, and raw nuts are optimal sources of the good kind of fats: monounsaturated and polyunsaturated.

- Regarding low sex drive: "One of the big culprits for both men and women is obesity. Their libido plummets due to biochemical changes that result in diminished blood flow. The extra weight also hinders their ability to have children....With Men it's damaged sperm; with women, it's ovulation problems."[4]

Back to my list of noticeable improvements in my lifestyle due to The Prehistoric Diet:

- Sinus and hay fever problems are 99% gone.

- Excellent digestion and regularity.

- No More Laryngitis

- Hair Growth: I have thicker hair and according to my research on hair growth, the following foods can contribute to this: sweet potatoes, melons, squash, carrots, apricots, fish and all seafood, eggs, raw nuts, seeds, all citrus fruits, berries, brussel sprouts, cauliflower, tomatoes, cucumbers, avocados, dark green leafy vegetables, whole grains, seaweed (many from Japan believe that seaweed is the secret to healthy hair), figs, asparagus, broccoli, lettuce, cabbage, poultry, and bananas.

Nutrition expert Michael Douney notes that "the more meat and fat a man eats, the higher his testosterone level and the more it converts within the hair follicles to dihydrotestosterone, which is basically follicle poison." Douney also notes that eating more vegetables and fruits can generally increase your chances of keeping your hair.[5]

- Better posture

- Much better state of mind; more positive; good attitude and spirits.

- Healthier looking skin

- Thinking faster, with more clarity

- Saving lots of money on my grocery bills:
  When you purchase highly packaged foods, which are highly advertised, you are paying for this advertising, which is many times more expensive than the cost of the actual food contents. In addition you are paying for all the other ingredients, i.e. the food additives. Also you are paying for the transportation of these products. Try to buy Produce from local produce stands

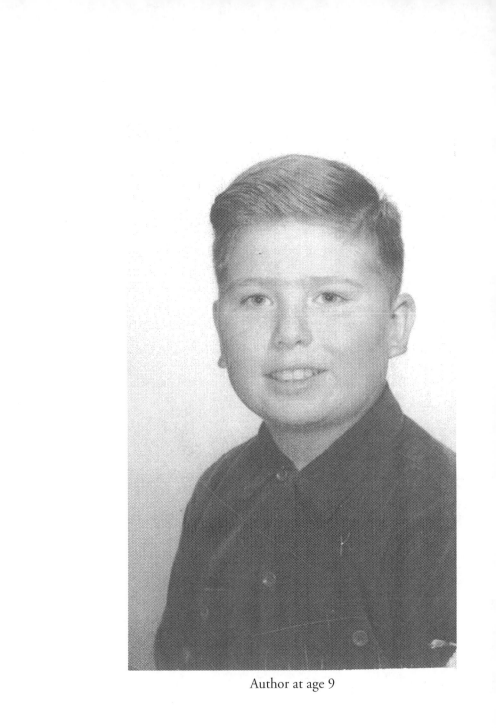

Author at age 9

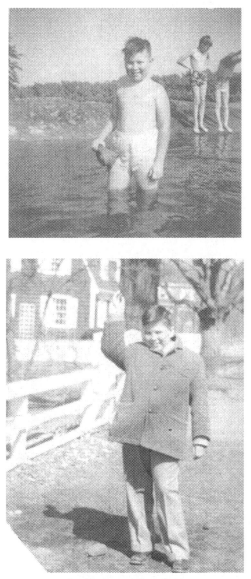

Author age 10 and 11
Chubby and smiling
(And not Happy)

4

A List of My "Friends"
(All The Wonderful Nature-Provided Foods)

And A List of Those That Are Not My Friends
(Foods that I Stay Away From)

My "Friends":

So you get hungry and are afraid that nature did not provide you with enough options. In fact, nature has provided plenty of wonderful options for you to choose from. Here's my list of "Friends". If any of these are problematic for you for some reason such as an allergy or are medically prohibited, then certainly omit them; there are still plenty of other foods to choose from. Remember: the great news is that you can eat as much

33

of these "Friends" as you want and whenever you want. Make sure you have lots on hand at home and that you take some to work so you never have to go without.

Please also note that everything on the list is to be as fresh as possible—not in cans (other than sardines) and not in packages unless frozen fruits and vegetables (make sure to read the ingredients to make sure there are no additives or unwanted elements. For instance if you buy a package of frozen blueberries, make sure the ingredients read just BLUEBERRIES and nothing else.).

FRUIT GROUP:

Pears

Grapefruit

Blueberries

Black raspberries

Strawberries

Cranberries

Mango

Cocoanut

Watermelon

Red Grapes

Purple Grapes

Green Grapes

Apples

Cherries

Guava

Tomatoes

Persimmon

Limes

Lemons

Oranges

Pineapple

Papaya

Tangerines

Nectarines

Peaches

Plums

Cantaloupe

Honeydew Melon

Figs (not dried)

Avocado

Bananas

VEGETABLE GROUP:

Watercress

Red cabbage

Green cabbage

Carrots

Yellow Bell Peppers

Green Bell Peppers

Red Bell Peppers

Green Hot Peppers

Broccoli

Zucchini

Butternut squash

Pumpkin

Acorn Squash

Boston Lettuce

Mushrooms

Celery

Brussel Sprouts

Seaweed

Sweet Potatoes

Parsnip

Beets

Red Onions

White Onions

Sweet Onions

Eggplant

Spaghetti Squash

Spinach

Baby Spinach

Romaine Lettuce

Boston Lettuce

Arugula

Radicchio

Radishes

Asparagus

Cucumbers

Artichokes

Mustard Greens

NUTS & SEEDS (All *raw* except chestnuts):

Cashews

Chestnuts

Pumpkin seeds

Sunflower seeds

Sesame seeds

Walnuts

Macadamia nuts

Pine Nuts

Filberts

Brazil Nuts

Almonds

Flax seeds

HERBS & SPICES:

Parsley

Tarragon

Dill

Mint

Cilantro

Thyme

Sage

Oregano

Sea Salt

Cinnamon

Basil

Scallions

Garlic

Ginger

Chives

HEAVY PROTEIN:

Chicken Breasts (no skin and make sure the chicken has no additives, hormones, colorings, etc.)

Turkey Breasts (same conditions as the chicken breast)

Lean Beef (no additives, should say grain-fed or vegetable-fed)

Venison (If possible)

Buffalo (If Possible)

Deep-water fish (should say WILD; do not buy farmed fish)

Salmon (Very important)

Tuna (not from a can)

Lobster (Not Farmed)

Shrimp (Not Farmed)

Scallops (Not Farmed)

All Shellfish (Not Farmed)

Sardines (If in a can, make sure in spring water)

BEVERAGES:

Water

Tea (All regular and herb teas)

Black coffee (Nice with cinnamon)

Freshly squeezed fruits juices

Freshly squeezed vegetable juices

Red wine (Cabernet Sauvignon, Pino Noir, Syrah)

OTHER FOODS:

Raw honey (Use sparingly)

Apple cider vinegar

Flax seed oil

Cod liver oil

Those that are NOT my "Friends":

Here is an explanation foods to avoid; they are NOT my "Friends". We have already established why it is important to stay away from the processed diet foods, drinks and soy. Any processed foods are a huge NO. The first processed foods occurred during the agricultural revolution about 10,000 years ago. Some on the list of "not my friends may surprise you but according to the "Prehistoric Diet" they are processed and are not meant for our nutrition as much as the wonderful foods established over 20 million years and provided for us by nature.

We, as humans, are part of the "animal kingdom" and as animals we graze. Nature meant for us to graze with her foods—foods not processed in any way. If you graze processed foods the results are horrendous—obesity, heart disease, diabetes, cancer etc.

The NO List

<u>No dairy foods of any kind</u>. Dairy foods are products of farming (the Agricultural Revolution). Dairy is a multi-billion dollar industry that has advertised for hundreds of years about the need for dairy. Our prehistoric ancestors knew about the only dairy needed. We have all heard the term "lactose intolerant," referring to those people that one cannot tolerate dairy products. These people become ill from dairy products.

The only milk needed for us humans is our mothers' milk at infancy. This is the way nature intended. A cow does not drink the milk of a camel and a camel does not drink the milk of a cat.

The question of course arises as to where to get our calcium. Where did our prehistoric ancestors get it?

Here are some great calcium sources: Green leafy vegetables, citrus fruits, raw nuts, broccoli, fish (sardines are a great source), eggshells, and meat with bone. Today we can have the above foods for calcium and there are calcium tablets at your natural food stores. Personally, I take egg shells (from boiled eggs, not raw) and grind them into a powder. Then I sprinkle the powder into my foods.

No Processed meats such as cold cuts.

No oils except flaxseed oil (flaxseed oil is a natural source of fiber and may be the best source of omega-3 fatty acids). Cod Liver oil is also excellent. All the processed oils make you put on weight, but luckily there are oils we can get from the good food list. We get oils from raw garlic, avocados, fish (salmon and sardines in particular) and raw nuts.

No margarine or mayonnaise

No Legumes (including peanuts, which are not nuts). Legumes put on weight and were utilized as a processed food during the Agricultural Revolution. While peanuts are a good source of nutrition, I prefer to find nutrition from the pre-agricultural revolution. It works for me.

<u>No white potatoes, pastas, or rice.</u>

<u>No pastries, energy bars, breads, candies or any sugars</u> other than those from the fruits and vegetables (and a little raw honey) on the "Friend" list

In the next chapter we will explore some recipes I've put together that work for me and many may work for you too. Before you know it, you too will be able to create your own wonderful "Prehistoric" life-enhancing and delicious recipes.

More good news: After a period of time on the "Prehistoric Diet," your body will be "turned off" to all the processed foods. You will cease to crave the bad stuff and you will always crave and "graze" the naturally needed and provided foods.

So go out and have fun...go explore...go graze...go grazy!

5

Recipe Ideas

These are some of my favorite recipes. The beauty of the Prehistoric Diet is that there is such an abundance of wonderful nature-provided foods that you will be your creative self and will be able think up your own recipes. Once you start exploring the possibilities, it can be pretty exciting. Please note that that the following recipes are intentionally ambiguous and contain no numbers or measurements. They are merely meant to get you thinking, so by all means mix and match ingredients and ratios as you please.

Beverages:

<u>Ice Coffee</u>: Black coffee with ice cubes and cinnamon. Try it in a wine goblet (somehow it's more fun that way). Make sure that the coffee is only coffee without any additives, sweeteners or flavorings.

Herb teas: Try the teas hot or chilled with a bit of raw honey and lemon juice if you wish

All Regular and Herbal Teas

Try the teas hot or chilled with a bit of Raw Honey and lemon juice if you wish

- Ginger Tea (Steep Sliced Ginger in hot water and add lemon juice)

- Cold ginger tea

Fresh water, with a squeeze of fresh lime juice or orange juice or lemon juice, in a wine goblet and on the rocks.

Freshly squeezed grapefruit or orange juice

Fresh vegetable juices (you will need a juicer for this)

Fruit smoothie: Berries, orange juice, cantaloupe, watermelon, peaches and any other fruits that appeals to you. Put in blender and liquefy.

Soups (Cold):

Gaspacho: Cut all in small pieces: Tomatoes, celery, red peppers, green peppers, parsley, chives, cilantro, mustard greens, cucumber, touch of lemon juice, touch of sea salt, touch of pepper. Put in blender to chop then chill.

Beet Borscht: Steamed Beets with some beet leaves, cucumber, lemon juice, chives, pinch of sea salt. Put in blender until smooth, then chill. Serve with a soft steamed parsnip or turnip in center.

Green Borscht: Cut up celery, parsley, radicchio, radish, spinach, chives, mustard greens and put in blender. Add a touch of apple cider vinegar, sea salt, and lemon juice. Blend on "blend" setting. Chill and serve with a ripe avocado in the center.

Sweet Soup: Cut up steamed sweet potatoes, beets, and carrots. Put in blender with cinnamon, a touch of water, touch of lemon juice, touch of sea salt. Blend until smooth and chill. Serve with a few leaves of mint on top.

Fruit soup: Berries, cantaloupe, peaches, add a touch of lime juice, blend until smooth and chill. Serve with a few leaves of mint on the center.

Cream of sweet potato soup: Steam sweet potatoes, cauliflower, and butternut squash. Boil some rolled oats. Put all in blender with cinnamon and nutmeg added, liquefy, chill and serve.

Soups (Hot):

Vegetable Soup: Cut up all your favorite vegetables, boil with sea salt to taste, lemon juice, some small pieces of garlic, and seaweed. Cook till all vegetables are medium soft.

Beef/Vegetable Soup: All the above plus lean beef, (cut in cubes). Sweet potatoes and onion are also really good to add in.

Tomato Soup: Cut up tomatoes, put in a blender with sea salt, pepper, lemon juice, blender at blend. Heat and stir. For a thicker soup, sprinkle in some rolled oats. Serve with a sliced avocado in the center

Sweet and Sour Soup: Cut sweet onions, red cabbage, beets, sweet potato, mustard leaves, and a few small pieces of ginger. Simmer till all is soft. Boil with sea salt and lemon juice.

Non-Dairy Creamed Soups: Boil cauliflower and rolled oats until soft. Put in blender with sea salt and lime or lemon juice until pureed. You can steam any of your favorite vegetables, beef, fish or chicken and use the broth. Mix in all together and warm up. A good non-dairy cream sauce is cauliflower and rolled oats blended together. Also good for creaminess is cooked spinach with avocado blended in. You can be very creative in how you use these combinations.

Grandma's Chicken Soup: Boil together chicken breasts (without the skin) or chicken cutlets, cut carrots, onion, celery, parsnip, a little garlic clove, a few pieces of ginger and turnip. Add in sea salt and lemon juice. Cook till chicken is cooked throughout and the vegetables are moderately soft.

Chicken and Rice (without rice) Soup: Do all the above but add in some steel cut oats which, when cooked, taste like rice.

Salads and Dressings:

Combinations for salads are unending and leave plenty of room for creativity. Here are some salads and dressings that I like:

Salad dressings:

- Apple cider vinegar mixed with sea salt, lime or lemon juice, flavored cod liver oil or flaxseed oil, pressed garlic

- Creamy salad dressing: take overripe avocado and mash in with apple cider vinegar, sea salt, and cooked rolled oats. Also add softly cooked cauliflower and flax seed oil or flavored cod liver oil.

- Mix fresh fruit juice such as orange, blueberry, strawberry with lemon juice, apple cider vinegar, flaxseed oil, and cut ginger.

Salads:

Beet Salad: Cut up boiled and chilled beets. Mix in with cut up sweet onions, a touch of oregano, cut up celery and cut up mushrooms.

Salad Nicoise: Assorted leafy green vegetables mixed in with a hard boiled egg, chilled cooked sweet potato, chilled cooked beets, sardines (packed in spring water), and baby carrots.

Cous Cous Salad: Mix cooked steel cut oats (cooled) with baby spinach and other greens, red onions, scallions, and sesame seeds.

Waldorf Salad: Assorted green leafy vegetables, mixed in with cut apples, walnuts, carrots, cucumbers, red onions.

Egg Salad: Hardboiled eggs, mixed in with flaxseed oil or flavored cod liver oil, cooked rolled oats, sea salt and lemon juice. Serve on Boston lettuce.

Mixed Fruit Salad: Cut up whatever fruits you want.

Side Dishes:

Guacamole: Mix ripe avocado, raw cut onions, pressed garlic, and sea salt. Blend and chill. Serve with as a topping to salad or pancakes or as a dip with fresh cut vegetables such as endives, celery sticks, vertically cut red peppers, and raw broccoli.

<u>Tsimmis</u>: Mix together cooked sweet potatoes, carrots, apples, pineapple, cinnamon, lemon juice, a touch of raw honey, and a touch of flaxseed oil.

<u>Ratatouille</u>: Mix cut up asparagus, tomatoes, carrots, onions, zucchini, ginger, lemon juice, sea salt, fresh oregano, sage and other herbs. Cook together with a little water.

<u>Baked Pancakes</u>: Blend together cooked steel cut oats, eggs, sea salt, onions and pressed garlic. Place on a cookie sheet with only a touch of flaxseed oil to grease the pan. Bake until the tops of the pancakes are firm then flip over. When baked, serve by itself or with a non-dairy cream sauce (see sauces).

<u>Baked Eggplant</u>: Cut eggplant into thin slices (about 1/4 inch thick), mix in rolled oats as well as egg and sea salt and other herbs. Dip the eggplant in the rolled oats and egg. Place on cookie sheet with a touch of flaxseed oil on sheet to grease the pan. Make sure the eggplant has the rolled oats on top. Bake until eggplant is soft, then flip over and make sure there are rolled oats and egg on the other side. Bake till all is cooked through and through. Top with a creamy (non-dairy) tomato sauce (see sauces).

Mixed Grilled Vegetables: Put thinly sliced vegetables such as beets, sweet potatoes, squash, and onions on a cookie sheet with a little water. Season with sea salt and lime juice and bake until soft on top. Flip over and cook till soft.

Seaweed: Mix dried seaweed with some apple cider vinegar and sesame seeds.

Dips & Sauces:

Creamy Tomato Sauce: Cook together tomatoes, cauliflower, and oatmeal. Add sea salt, oregano and other herbs, as well as a touch of lemon juice. Blend till smooth. Good on chicken, baked eggplant and baked pancakes.

Non-Dairy Cream Sauce: Mix cooked eggplant, oatmeal, cauliflower, with sea salt, lime or lemon juice, and a touch of flaxseed oil. Blend till smooth. Good on fish.

Salsa: Mix cut onions, celery, tomatoes, cilantro, sea salt, small pieces of garlic, and apple cider vinegar. Serve with baked pancakes or with endives to dip.

Non-Dairy Creamed Green Sauce: Mix cooked spinach, cooked oatmeal, ripened avocado, and cooked cauliflower. Add sea salt and limejuice. Blend till smooth. Good on chicken and fish.

Creamed Beet and Squash Sauce: Mix cooked spinach and cooked butternut squash. Add sea salt, some flaxseed oil, and lemon juice. Blend till smooth. Good on fish.

Entrees:

Ginger/Garlic Chicken: Prepare chicken breasts without the skin. Make slits and put in small slivers of garlic and ginger. Sprinkle with a little sea salt. Bake till the chicken is half done and then turn over. Bake till done.

Poached Egg with Seaweed: Put about ½" of water in a frying pan and heat till boiled. Gently break egg yolks into the water. When the eggs look firm turn over till eggs are fully cooked. Place seaweed on plate and place poached egg on seaweed. Sprinkle sea salt, a touch of lime juice and sesame seeds on top.

Beef Stew: Try to purchase lean beef cubes that have no additives. Better yet, try to find vegetable-fed beef. Simmer the beef with cut sweet potatoes, carrots, mushrooms, steel cut oats, onions, turnips, parsnip and a few cut cloves of garlic and parsley. Season with sea salt and lemon juice. Simmer till all vegetables are soft and the beef is cooked to medium rare.

Rolled Oat Fish Almandine: Mix egg and rolled oats with some sea salt and lemon juice. Dip the fish in the mixture then place on the cookie sheet. Make sure that the mixture covers the entire fish. Bake till top looks cooked then turn over and sprinkle some cut up raw almonds and a sprig of thyme on the other side. Cook till done.

Sweet & Sour Baked Fish: Place fish on cookie sheet, sprinkle on lemon juice and sea salt. Place sliced apples on top of the fish along with dark (pitted) cherries and oregano. Bake till done on both sides.

Chicken and Steel Cut Oats: Boil a good portion of steel cut oats with chicken cutlets. Add sea salt, lemon juice, oregano, carrots, mushrooms, and some garlic gloves. Cook till chicken and vegetables are cooked through. Let stand on pot for a while so all the juices marinate a bit. When ready to plate, add some flaxseed oil and mix in.

Soufle: put 1/4 of inch of water in frying pan to a full boil mix in a bowl 3 eggs, a handful of steel cut oats, cut vegetables, seasonings. Put in frying pan and turn over all till it is firm.

Desserts:

Fresh fruits make for the best desserts. Please note that if you add a few drops of fresh lemon juice to your fruit (especially melon), it will enhance the sweetness. Here are some other ideas and variations:

Half-Frozen Grapes: Wash some seedless grapes and put in the freezer. When half frozen, take out. Note the sorbet-like taste; the freezing enhances the sweetness.

Sweet Potato Pudding: Put baked sweet potato in blender with cooked rolled oats, fresh mango, fresh pineapple, and a touch of lemon juice. Blend and freeze till chilled. Top with a peppermint leaf.

Very Orange Custard: Mix baked sweet potato, orange, very ripe cantaloupe, cooked butternut squash, baby carrots, cooked rolled oats, and ripe banana. Blend all and chill in freezer. Top with cinnamon and nutmeg.

Baked Apple: Cut apples in half, top with cinnamon and a bit of lemon juice. Bake till soft.

Apple Sauce: Cut apples and core them, removing the seeds. Boil in ½ " of water. When apples are soft, put in blender with cinnamon and a bit of lemon juice.

Sorbets: Look for bags of frozen fruits at your local grocery store. It is usually fairly easy to find frozen blueberries, strawberries, blackberries, raspberries, dark cherries, and mango. Make sure the contents are fruits only. Defrost at room temperature till soft. Blend with some lemon juice and then freeze till almost frozen.

Banana Custard: Mash up banana with lots of cinnamon, some cooked rolled oats, and some fresh orange juice. Add some coconut milk. Put in freezer till half-frozen.

Berries N' Oats: Mix hot cooked steel-cut oats, adding lots of frozen blueberries, cinnamon, and just a touch of honey.

<u>Smoothies</u>: Cut into small pieces banana, any fruits, carrots, and ginger. Add crushed ice. Put in blender.

Snacks Away from Home:

Once you have been on The Prehistoric Diet for a certain amount time (which varies according to the individual), you will no longer be enticed by the NO list. Your body will simply be turned off to it. As mentioned, we are animals meant to graze, so here are some ideas for snacks while away from home:

- Raw nuts

- Raw sunflower seeds

- Celery sticks

- Baby carrots

- Fresh fruit

- Water

- Iced coffee, black with cinnamon

6

Summary

"If I am not for myself, who will be for me? And if I am
only for myself, what am I? And if not now, when?"

-Rabbi Hillel

A little pep talk.

We ourselves and many people we know have
struggled with weight issues. They have tried gyms and
purchasing of expensive exercise machines, popped diet
pills, as well as hyped-up media weight plans, only to put
the weight back on, many times ending up worse off than
before.

Nature took 20,000,000 years to perfect The
Prehistoric Diet for you, the perfect being. Take it, use
it—it is yours to keep. Follow this and you will never be
overweight or obese again. You will add years to your life
and will feel years younger.

We are bombarded with media and merchandising hype to sell us products that are making us sicker and poorer. We see advertisements for these products on television, on billboards, and in magazines. We watch cooking shows, pop weight loss pills, and see glittering food ads galore.

It can sometimes seem impossible to surmount all of this, but we can and we must fight back. We are not sheep; we do not follow; **"We lead ourselves to become ourselves"**

Here are some of the things we can do:

1. **Nutrition begins in our home.**

    I suggest that, immediately after reading and understanding The Prehistoric Diet, go through *all* your food shelves and your fridge and "dump the junk." Go to your grocery stores and purchase the foods on the food lists given in chapter 4 and refer to the recipes in chapter 5 for further ideas and encouragement. Fill up your home with these foods and eat them whenever you want and as much as you want. You will never be hungry and very soon you will start to reap the benefits.

    We are all familiar with "comfort food," which many of us rely upon in order to deal with stress. Well, eat away! But eat *only* what you have in your home. As you see the weight come off, you will begin feeling better. Chances are some of your stress will be alleviated and you'll be eating less before you know it.

    Just be sure to "lay down the law" to yourself and your family. Make it clear to yourself and your loved ones that this is the way it is: no more junk is to enter the home. Period.

2. **Work with your schools, school boards and PTA's to ensure better foods and nutrition in your schools cafeterias.**

Here's an interesting note: A school in Miami Beach, Florida showed that by improving the nutrition of school meals, academic performance greatly improved and, after a period of time, the students lost weight and had lower blood pressure. The study also showed how excited the children were about the better nutrition, the higher self esteem they felt and that they actually loved fiber and broccoli.

Also, the advocacy group *The Cancer Project* has criticized school lunch menus for including processed meats such as hotdogs and deli meats on their menus. Such meats are linked to colorectal cancer. This study was done in 29 U.S. school districts. Only districts in San Francisco and Denver were judged as satisfactory.[1]

Have seminars in the schools about the Prehistoric Diet, put up posters in the cafeterias about better nutrition. Get as many foods as possible from the Prehistoric Diet as part of the cafeteria meals. Have essay contests about nutrition. Have "Prehistoric" Food Fairs.

3. **Organize!**

If you live in an area where you feel the grocery stores do not have the wonderful foods that you desire and it is a hardship to shop outside your area, then band together with your neighbors and go en masse to your local food stores to let them know that you will only shop there if the "good foods" are there for you to purchase. Trust me—grocery stores will respond.

4. **Work** with your city and town governments to put pressure on all fast food stores near the schools. Demand that they offer a lot of wonderful "Good Foods" and, better yet, encourage fruit and vegetable stands near every school possible so your children have options right near them.

5. **Use chop sticks at home.** It's fun, and you may eat less since it take more time to eat. Many studies show that children increase their dexterity by using chop sticks.

6. **Drink** a glass of water before meals or snacks. Water (especially with lemon juice) is a cleanser and will help to fill you up.

7. When you start losing weight, get rid of your "fat" clothes or go to a tailor and take them in.

8. **Ordering at Restaurants: Is this a problem?**
   Not really. I personally enjoy knowing how the foods are prepared that I take into my body so the next best thing to eating at home is to be very particular about where you eat and what and

how you order. Choose a restaurant where you feel there is quality food. Do not be intimidated when ordering and try to adhere as closely as possible to the Prehistoric Diet. Ask for no dairy, no oils, and no starches. Remember: You are a paying customer; you are in control.

9. It is often said that we are only as good as our surroundings, often meaning places and people. Try to socialize with people who encourage your Prehistoric way of eating and, even better, develop a circle of friends and relatives that are also with you on this miraculous journey of health strength and wonderful life. Try to stay away from those that will try to discourage you. It is your health and your body.

As a precaution, I must state again that if there are certain food allergies that you have then certainly stay away from those foods. Also, if you are on certain medications then I certainly do not advise you to discontinue them. I do, however, advise anyone to investigate what their medications are all about as far as benefits and side effects. I personally feel that if we are able to do without medications, we will be better off because of it.

IN CONCLUSION, I would like to thank our prehistoric ancestors for helping to develop their diet, and most certainly the heavens above for providing us with all the natural foods within our environment and the intelligence to use them. **It took 20 million years.**

References

Chapter 1

[1] "New York Post" July 18 2008: Source: Center for Disease Control and Prevention

[2] Health Section "Metro" NYC September 8, 2008

[3] (CDC); Kim O'Donnel "The Washington Post"

Chapter 2

[1] Deborah Kotz "US News & World Report"

[2] "San Francisco Chronicle" January 2006. Environment California.org

[3] www.niehs.nih.gov/news/media/questions/sya-bpa.cfm 8/23/2008

[4] *Ibid.*

[5] "The EPOCH" (VOA News).

[6] George Fredericks Pharmacy Director/Albany N.Y. Hospital Group Oct 14 2007 Stephanie Earls, Albany Times Union

[7] Jay Lindsay Associated Press writer

[8] Dr. Jay Mazzella of Gallagher Chiroprobetic Leonardo NY. Diet Soda—Less Calories, more side effects 3-1-08

[9] Morando Soffritti Fiorelli Belpoggi; Davide Degli Esposti,Luco Lambertini Cancer Research Center. European Ramazzini Foundation, Oncology and Environmental Sciences, Bologna Italy

[10] Olney J.W.etcel; Increasing Brain Tumor Rates: Journal of Neuropathology and Experimental Neurology Vol.55, No11 November 1996

[11] www.dorway.com/badnews.html

[12] Janet Starr Hull Creator of the Aspartame Detox Program

[13] McMan's Depression and Bipolarweb 2008

[14] June 25 2007: Consumer Service Protection Institute

[15] 11/17/99 MSDNYMBER:C4730 Mallinckrodt&Baker Inc

[16] WIKI ANSWERS 2008

[17] "EPOCH" New York (Reuters)

[18] Website Rung International an iso 9001 company

[19] American Heritage Dictionary

[20] Judith Shaw "Raising Low Fat Kids in a High Fat World"

[21] Hydrogenated Oils-Silent Killers by Columnist David Lawrence Dewey. Copyright 1996

[22] Underhill et al 1929

[23] Spencer Lender 1979

[24] "Wall Street Journal" column by Michael Waldholz Feb 20 2003

[25] Copyright 1996-2006 Cerner Multum Inc. 2-`14-07

[26] Columbia Encyclopedia Sixth Edition 2008

[27] Copyright 1996-2008 Cerner Multum Inc. 4-25-08

[28] "Body Active Online"

[29] Copyright 2006-2008 Daisy House INC.

[30] Michael Pollick copyright 2003-2008 Conjecture Corporation

[31] www.fdu.gov/bbs/topics/consumer/lonov259.htm/

[32] MSDS Number F1802 5-4-07

[33] Who Food Additives Series 142 Genera 1999 IPCS-International Programs on Chemical Safety

[34] "Amy's Kitchen" Feb 27 2007 Mike Adams

[35] NANO FOODS: The Next Consumer Scare?" "EPOCH " New York. 8-7-08 Science and technology

[36] Rackis,Joseph J.etal;"The USDA Trypsin Inhibitor Study I. Backround Objections and Procedures details "Qualifications of Plant Foods In Human Nutrition, Vol.351985

[37] The Weston A. Price Foundation for Wise Traditions Studies Showing Adverse Effects of Dictory Soy 1975-2003

[38] ISHIZUKI, et al. "The Effects on the Thyroid Gland of Soybeans Administered experimentally in healthy subjects" Nippon Naibunpi Gakkai Zasshi (1991) 967-622-629

Chapter 3

[1] Eaton SB.Eatonsb11, Konnes M Jeal Journal of Nutrition June 1996: 126:1732-40

[2] Epoch Times June 4,2008 Dr. John Briffa

[3] New Hope Blog.com

[4] Men's Health Feb 6 2008

[5] Michael Russell Ezire Articles.com

Chapter 5

[1] AMNY.Com/health Sept 24.08 "Bad News for School Lunch" U.S. News & World Report